# SELF-CONTROL
# A GATEWAY TO ULTIMATE HAPPINESS

True happiness begins where self-control takes root.

By

**JIVANAM**

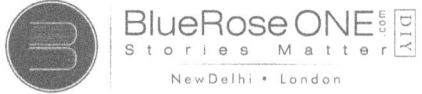

**BLUEROSE PUBLISHERS**
India | U.K.

Copyright © Jivanam 2025

All rights reserved by author. No part of this publication may be reproduced, stored in a retrieval system or transmitted in any form or by any means, electronic, mechanical, photocopying, recording or otherwise, without the prior permission of the author. Although every precaution has been taken to verify the accuracy of the information contained herein, the publisher assumes no responsibility for any errors or omissions. No liability is assumed for damages that may result from the use of information contained within.

BlueRose Publishers takes no responsibility for any damages, losses, or liabilities that may arise from the use or misuse of the information, products, or services provided in this publication.

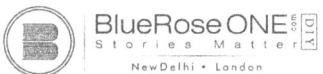

For permissions requests or inquiries regarding this publication,
please contact:

BLUEROSE PUBLISHERS
www.BlueRoseONE.com
info@bluerosepublishers.com
+91 8882 898 898
+4407342408967

ISBN: 978-93-7139-815-2

First Edition: June 2025

**Dedication**

To every soul striving to rise above impulse and live with clarity.

May you discover the quiet strength within, and the joy that follows.

# Table of Contents

Preface – 1

Author's Message – 2

Introduction – 3

## Part 1: Understanding Self-Control

1. The Happiness Myth – 5

2. Redefining Self-Control – 12

3. The Science of Self-Control – 18

4. Freedom Through Discipline – 25

## Part 2: Mastering Mind & Emotions

5. Emotional Intelligence – 32

6. The Art of Delayed Gratification – 38

7. Breaking Addictions – 45

8. Training Your Thoughts – 52

## Part 3: Self-Control in Daily Life

9. Mastering Habits – 61

10. The Power of Routine – 68

11. Self-Control in Relationships – 75

12. Financial Self-Control – 81

## Part 4: The Ultimate Reward – True Happiness

13. The Joy of Saying No – 88

14. Mindfulness & Self-Control – 94

15. Redefining Success – 100

16. Your Journey Forward – 106

## Preface

We live in a world of constant stimulation
where every urge demands instant attention, and pleasure
often masquerades as happiness.

This book was born from a quiet realization:
that true joy doesn't come
from getting everything we want, but
from mastering the mind that wants it all.

"Self-Control - A Gateway to Ultimate Happiness"
is not a theory-heavy text, nor a list of rigid rules.
It's a mirror - gently reflecting the power
you already hold within.

If you're ready to reclaim your attention, calm your
emotions, and find freedom through discipline, this book is
your invitation.

May these pages serve as
your guide – not toward perfection, but toward
presence, purpose, and peace.

## Author's Message

Dear Reader,

This book is designed as a practical guide - a diary of essential points - to help you navigate life with greater clarity, awareness, and balance. Think of it as a companion that you can return to whenever real-life situations challenge your inner stability. Refer to the relevant sections, reflect deeply, and allow the insights to guide you toward making wise, composed decisions. With time and practice, you'll find that your self-control strengthens, empowering you to take charge of your life more effectively.

I warmly encourage you to move through this book slowly - one chapter at a time. Give each concept the space it deserves in your mind. Let the ideas simmer, churn, and settle until your doubts and questions begin to resolve themselves. This process of deep internalization is what brings true clarity and lasting transformation.

My heartfelt wish is that you grow, express your highest potential, and live your life to its fullest with ultimate happiness.

With gratitude,

**Jivanam**

## Introduction

What if happiness wasn't something to chase – but something you could cultivate from within?

In a world full of distractions, instant gratification, and pressure to perform, self-control isn't just a virtue - it's a superpower.

*"Self-Control – A Gateway to Ultimate Happiness"* offers a practical and powerful roadmap to reclaim your time, attention, and energy.

Through science, timeless wisdom, and real-world insights, this book will help you:

- Master your impulses
- Strengthen emotional clarity
- Build lasting habits
- Improve relationships
- Find peace in the present moment

If you're ready to live with more intention, resilience, and authentic joy - start here.

# PART -1

## Understanding Self-Control

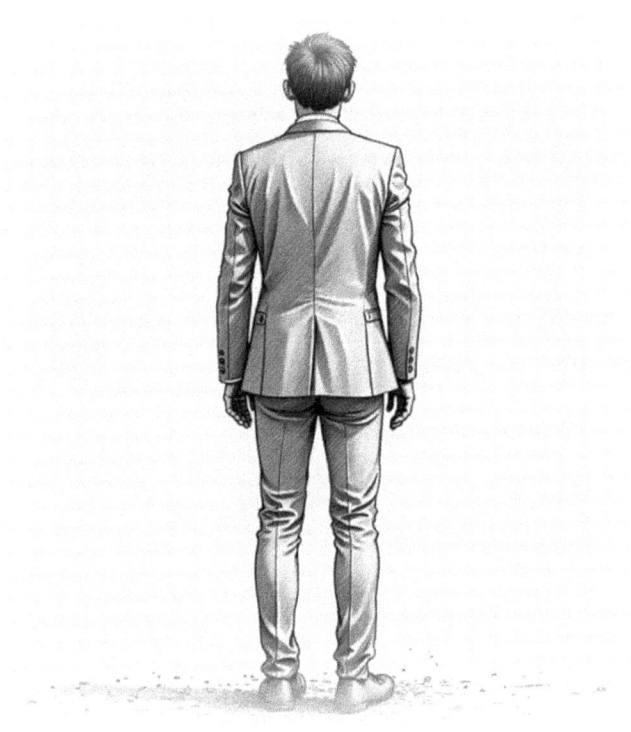

# Chapter 1

# The Happiness Myth –

# Why Pleasure Isn't Enough

In today's fast-paced world, happiness is often sold to us in shiny packaging - a new phone, a decadent dessert, a thrilling vacation, or a viral video. Modern culture has subtly trained us to believe that the key to happiness lies in pleasure - the more, the better. We chase it, accumulate it, and measure our lives by how much of it we can experience. But despite the abundance of pleasures available at our fingertips, many still find themselves feeling empty, restless, or even unhappy. Why?

This chapter uncovers the myth that pleasure equals happiness and explains why true, lasting happiness lies elsewhere - in something deeper, more meaningful, and surprisingly powerful: self-control.

**The Pursuit of Pleasure**

Let's start with what pleasure really is. Pleasure is a response - a temporary emotional high that our brain rewards us with when we experience something enjoyable. Eating a sweet treat, buying something new, watching your favorite show - all this trigger the brain's reward system, especially a chemical called **dopamine**.

Now, there's nothing wrong with pleasure itself. It's natural and necessary. However, when we start equating pleasure with happiness, we fall into a trap. Because pleasure is fleeting, and the moment it fades, we seek it again. This creates a cycle - a loop of constant chasing without ever feeling truly satisfied.

This phenomenon is what psychologists refer to as the **"hedonic treadmill"**. You keep running, expecting to arrive at happiness, but you stay in the same place emotionally. You might get the raise, the car, the applause - but then your mind resets, and the chase begins again.

**The False Promise of Instant Gratification**

Pleasure offers quick rewards, which is why instant gratification is so tempting. You feel a craving, and you act on it. But over time, this pattern reduces our capacity for patience, resilience, and discipline - traits that are essential for long-term happiness and fulfillment.

Think about the satisfaction that comes from:

- Finishing a big project
- Learning a new skill
- Overcoming a challenge

These experiences require effort and perseverance - often without immediate pleasure - yet they give us a deep sense of pride and joy. That's the difference between pleasure and fulfillment. One fades quickly, the other builds lasting contentment.

## The Wisdom of Ancient Traditions

Interestingly, ancient wisdom has always pointed to this truth. From the Stoic philosophers of Greece to the teachings of the Bhagavad Gita in India, self-control and inner mastery have been praised as keys to a meaningful life.

The Buddha taught that craving is the root of suffering. Socrates believed the unexamined life isn't worth living, implying that reflection and self-awareness matter more than indulgence. In the Gita, Krishna advises Arjuna to act with discipline and detachment, rather than being driven by pleasure or pain.

These teachings don't deny pleasure - they just don't worship it. Instead, they emphasize something more enduring: self-control, purpose, and inner peace.

## Why Pleasure Alone Can't Sustain Happiness

**Let's break it down:**

1. **Pleasure is temporary.** It disappears as quickly as it comes.
2. **It creates dependency.** We often need more and more to feel the same level of joy.
3. **It distracts from deeper needs.** When we seek quick fixes and easy highs, we unknowingly put our true growth on hold. Physical strength, mental clarity, and emotional resilience are built through patience, not instant gratification.

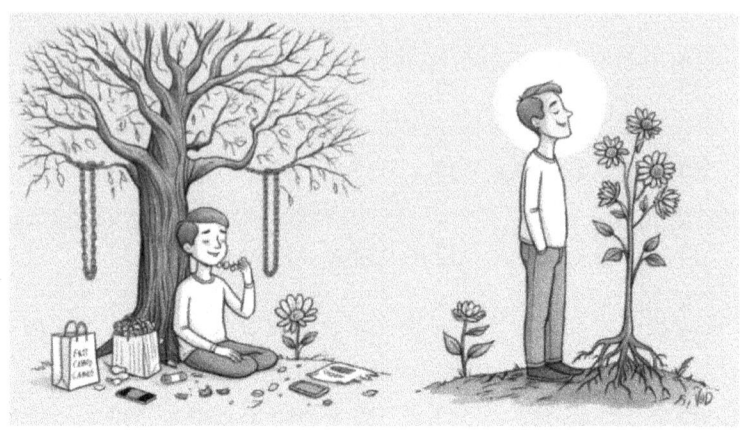

4. **It can lead to guilt or regret.** Especially when it becomes compulsive - like overeating, overspending, or excessive screen time.

True happiness, on the other hand, is rooted in meaning, purpose, and self-mastery. It's about becoming the kind of person you're proud of, living with intention, and feeling aligned with your values.

**The Shift: From Chasing to Choosing**

The moment you stop chasing pleasure and start choosing purpose, something profound happens. You begin to experience a different kind of happiness - one that isn't based on circumstances but on character. A calm satisfaction, a sense of strength and a quiet joy that doesn't scream for attention but glows from within.

This shift requires self-control. It requires the ability to pause, to say no when necessary, and to act in line with your long-term well-being rather than short-term desires.

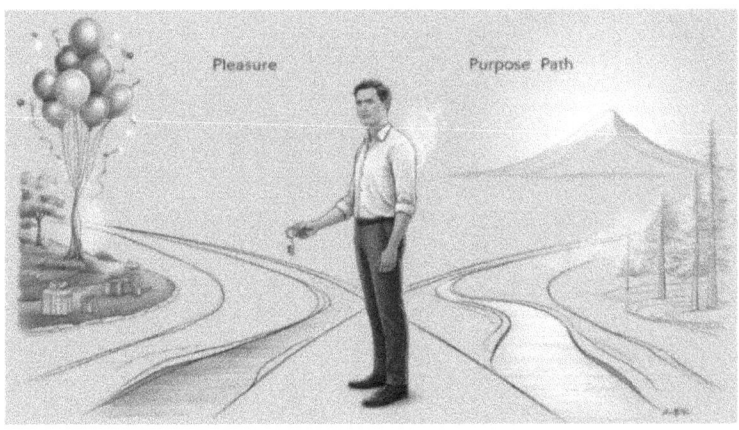

**Self-control doesn't mean denying yourself everything** or living a joyless life. Quite the opposite. It means becoming the master of your mind and your choices - and in doing so, unlocking a deeper kind of joy.

**A Real-Life Example: The Ice Cream Dilemma**

After a long and exhausting day at work, Albert came home feeling drained. As he walked into his kitchen, the freezer light caught his eye. Inside was his favorite ice cream- smooth, sweet, and comforting. Without thinking much, he grabbed it, flopped onto the couch, and started eating. For a few minutes, it felt good. The stress seemed to melt away with each bite. But soon, the tiredness returned-this time with a hint of emptiness he couldn't explain.

Just across the street, Billy had a day just as tiring. But when he got home, something different greeted him-his dog Max, tail wagging and full of excitement. Billy smiled. He knelt down, played fetch for a while, and laughed as Max jumped around with joy. It wasn't anything big, but it made him feel genuinely better. When Billy finally walked inside, his body was still tired, but his heart was lighter. Not because he escaped his stress, but because he chose something real and joyful.

There's a quiet truth in these two stories:

Albert found quick comfort that didn't last. Billy found joy that filled him from the inside out.

The small choices we make in our low moments often shape the bigger picture of our lives.

Most of us, truthfully, are like Albert. We look for quick fixes-snacks, screens, scrolling. Few of us are like Billy, who choose connection, presence, and small actions that lift us up from the inside.

Now imagine this: instead of reaching for a quick escape, you pause. You take a deep breath and choose something just a little better-like a short walk, your favorite music, a cold shower, a stretch, or journaling your thoughts for ten minutes.

In that pause, something powerful happens. You're not reacting anymore. You're responding. And that simple act of self-control doesn't just give you short-term comfort-it gives you pride, clarity, and strength.

That's where real change begins,
When you feel the pull... pause... and choose something that truly supports you-not just for a moment, but for the long run.

**The Beginning of Real Joy**

This chapter is the doorway to the rest of your journey. By understanding the limits of pleasure, you can begin to open yourself to something richer. The kind of happiness that doesn't depend on things going your way, but on you becoming your best self – self rooted in clarity, calm, and control.

In the coming chapters, we'll dive into how to build this self-control - mentally, emotionally, and practically - so you can start living with more focus, peace, and fulfillment.

You deserve more than momentary pleasure.

You deserve lasting happiness - and it begins with reclaiming your inner power.

# Chapter 2

# Redefining Self-Control – More Than Just Willpower

When we hear the word **self-control**, most people picture gritting their teeth, resisting temptation, and forcing themselves to do something they don't feel like doing. This narrow view associates it with **willpower** - a mental muscle we're either born with or not. However, self-control is not just about resisting what's bad; it's about creating space for what's truly good.

In this chapter, we'll broaden the definition of self-control. You'll learn why it's more than just saying "no," and how it's actually the foundation of **freedom**, **clarity**, and **confidence**.

### The Common Misunderstanding

Let's face it, self-control has a bad reputation.

People often think:

- "It's **boring**."
- "It's for **perfectionists** or monks."
- "It takes the **fun** out of life."

But this view is misleading. It paints self-control as restrictive, even painful - something you use only when forced to, like a punishment for being human.

In truth, self-control isn't about punishment - it's about **empowerment**. It's not about deprivation - it's about liberation from impulses and distractions that steal your time, energy, and peace.

Think of it this way:

**Self-control** isn't about suppressing who you are. It's about shaping who you become.

## Willpower Has Limits

There's no denying that willpower plays a role in self-control, but it's only one piece of the puzzle. Willpower is like a battery - it gets depleted with overuse. That's why it's hard to make healthy choices at the end of a long, stressful day when your mental energy is drained.

Studies show that willpower is:

- Finite - it weakens with fatigue, stress, and decision overload.
- Fragile - emotional disturbances, distractions, or low blood sugar can reduce it.
- Unreliable - it fluctuates daily depending on sleep, mood, and routine.

So, if self-control was only about brute-force willpower, most of us would fail daily. But the good news is - it's not.

## A Better Definition of Self-Control

Let's redefine self-control in a more accurate and empowering way:

**Self-control** is the conscious ability to align your actions with your inner values and goals - even when it's hard.

It's a skill, a mindset, and a quiet inner strength that grows with practice.

This redefinition opens up new doors. Self-control is not something you either have or don't; it's something you build. It's a system you can design, and it's not about resisting life - it's about living intentionally.

## The Three Pillars of Self-Control

To truly master self-control, you need more than willpower. You need a strong foundation. Think of it as a structure supported by **three pillars**:

1. **Awareness**: You can't control what you're not aware of. Self-control begins with noticing your impulses, emotions, and triggers. It's about developing mindfulness and catching yourself before acting on autopilot.

2. **Values & Vision**: What are you aiming for? Self-control becomes easier when you're clear about your goals, values, and the kind of person you want to be. Without a vision, control feels like suffering. With a vision, it becomes purpose.

3. **Systems & Habits**: Discipline doesn't always have to be hard - it can be automatic. If you create smart systems (like morning routines, digital boundaries, or meal prep), you rely less on willpower and more on structure.

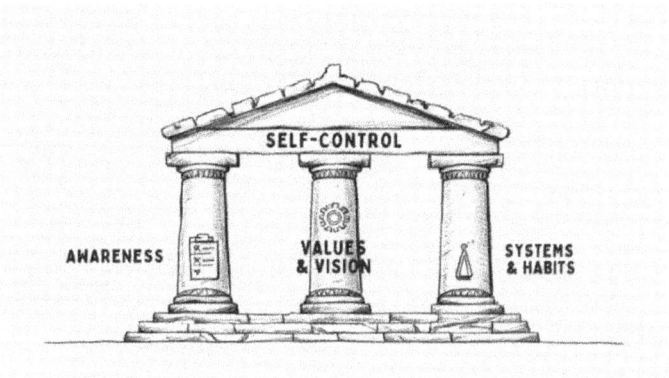

**Self-Control Is Freedom in Disguise**

Here's a paradox worth remembering:

**Discipline leads to freedom.**

At first glance, that seems backwards. Isn't freedom doing whatever you want, whenever you want?

But real freedom - the kind that matters - isn't about doing everything. It's about doing the right things and being free from regret, guilt, anxiety, or addiction.

- **The person who controls their money** isn't restricted - they're free from debt.
- **The one who controls their emotions** isn't cold - they're free from chaos.

- **The one who controls their attention** isn't boring - they're free from distraction.

Self-control gives you the power to choose your future, instead of being pulled by your impulses.

**Self-Control Is Not Self-Denial**

It's important to draw the line between self-control and self-denial.

**Self-denial** says: "You can't have that. Ever."

**Self-control** says: "You can have that - but not at the cost of your peace, goals, or health."

It's not about saying "no" to everything - it's about saying "yes" to what truly matters.

A person with self-control doesn't fear pleasure - they just don't let pleasure control them. They enjoy dessert, but they're not ruled by sugar. They take a break, but they don't avoid responsibility. They live balanced, intentional lives.

**Real-Life Scenario: The Phone Habit**

Let's say you have a habit of checking your phone every few minutes. You tell yourself to stop. You try using willpower. Maybe it works for a day, then you relapse.

But what if you redefined the problem?

- First, you become aware: You realize you check your phone when you're bored or anxious.
- Then, you remember your values: You want to be more present, focused, and less reactive.

- Finally, you design a system: You turn off notifications, use a time-limiter app, and keep your phone in another room during work hours.

Now, self-control isn't just you fighting a craving. It's you, shaping your environment and behavior to align with who you want to be. That's real power.

---

**Final Thoughts**

Redefining self-control is essential to reclaiming your life. When you see it as a painful force of will, you avoid it. But when you see it as a skill that helps you live on purpose, everything changes.

Self-control isn't the enemy of joy - it's the pathway to real joy. It's not the opposite of freedom - it's how you protect and expand your freedom. And it's not about saying no forever - it's about saying yes to the best version of yourself.

In the next chapter, we'll explore what science has discovered about the brain's role in self-control and how you can use it to your advantage.

Your power isn't in resisting life.

Your power is in shaping it.

# Chapter 3

# The Science of Self-Control – How Your Brain Works

You now understand that self-control is more than just willpower - it's about awareness, structure, and aligning your actions with your values. To master self-control, it helps you to know what's happening inside your brain when you feel tempted, distracted, or impulsive.

This chapter takes you inside the human brain, where self-control is born, tested, and strengthened. Understanding this gives you an incredible advantage: you can work with your brain instead of constantly fighting against it.

**The Battle Inside Your Brain**

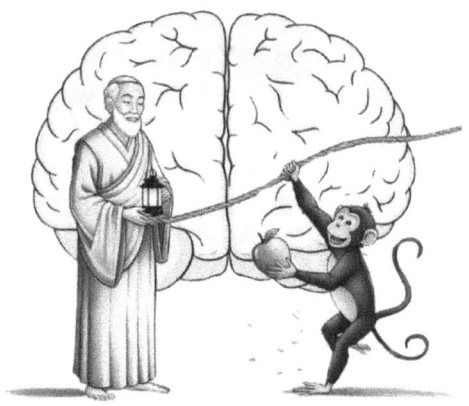

Your brain is a beautifully complex organ, but when it comes to decision-making and self-control, it helps to think of it as two parts in constant conversation:

1. The Prefrontal Cortex – the **rational thinker**

Located behind your forehead, this part of the brain is responsible for planning, long-term thinking, impulse control, and decision-making. It's the "wise guide" - the part of you that says, "Let's go to bed early because we have an early morning."

2. The Limbic System – the **emotional reactor**

Deep in the brain lies a more primitive system, including the amygdala and nucleus accumbens, which controls emotion, reward, and cravings. It's the part that screams, "Eat that cake now!" or "Check your phone again - maybe there's a message!"

Self-control is essentially the ongoing dialogue between these two parts. Your higher brain wants long-term gain. Your emotional brain wants instant reward. Learning to manage this tug-of-war is the essence of self-mastery.

**The Dopamine Factor**

Let's talk about **dopamine**, often called the brain's "pleasure chemical." But that's only part of the story. Dopamine is not just about feeling good - it's about anticipation. It gets released when your brain expects a reward.

Every time you get a notification, a sugary snack, or a win in a video game, your brain gives you a hit of dopamine. It trains your behaviour by rewarding certain actions - even if those actions aren't aligned with your goals.

This is why so many people get stuck in habit loops:

Trigger → Craving → Action → Reward (Example of Instagram habit loop)

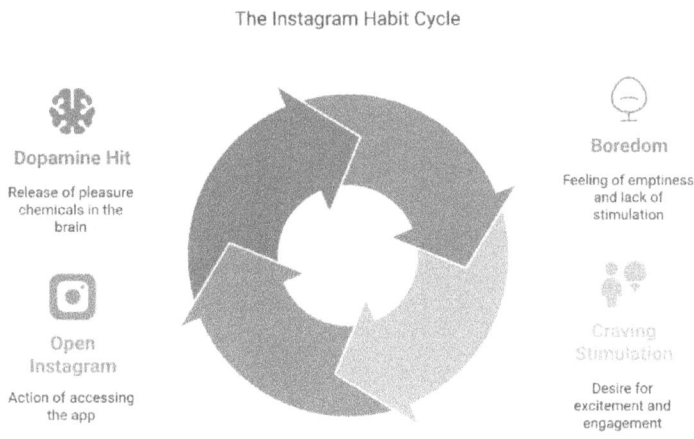

Over time, your brain wires itself to expect that reward. Unless you rewire those circuits, it becomes increasingly hard to break the cycle.

**Neuroplasticity: You're Not Stuck**

Here's the good news: your brain is not fixed.

Thanks to something called **neuroplasticity**, your brain is capable of changing itself - creating new pathways and habits through repetition and conscious effort.

Every time you resist a distraction, pause before reacting, or choose a healthy behaviour, you're strengthening the neural connections in your prefrontal cortex. You're literally rewiring your brain for better self-control.

Think of your mind like a jungle trail. The more you walk the same path, the clearer it becomes. The less you use an old path, the more it gets overgrown. With daily practice, your default behaviour can change.

**Stress: The Silent Saboteur**

Stress is one of the biggest enemies of self-control. When you're under pressure, your brain shifts resources away from the rational prefrontal cortex and gives control to the emotional brain - the survival system.

That's why people often:

- Eat junk food after a hard day.
- Lash out in anger during arguments.
- Procrastinate when feeling overwhelmed.

Stress makes short-term relief feel like the only option. Managing stress is essential for maintaining self-control.

**Key Tip:** Build in micro-recovery moments throughout your day.

Try these simple, powerful habits:

- **Set an hourly reminder.** Just a gentle nudge to pause, breathe, and reset your focus. Even 30 seconds can change your mindset.

- **Drink a glass of water every hour.** Hydration fuels both your body and mind. It's a small act of care that grounds you.

- **Take three deep breaths.** Let them be slow and intentional. It helps calm your nervous system and brings you back to the present.

- **Feel gratitude.** In one quiet moment, reflect on something you're thankful for: your breath, your home, your loved ones, even the chance to start fresh.

- **Go for a short walk.** Even five minutes of movement outside can lift your mood and shake off mental fog.

- **Break your environment.** Step away from your screen. Change rooms. Look at the sky. Let your mind breathe.

**Sleep, Nutrition & Self-Control**

Your brain is a physical organ. Its ability to function - including making good decisions - depends on how well you take care of your body.

- Sleep: Lack of sleep weakens the prefrontal cortex and increases emotional reactivity. Even one bad night can make self-control harder the next day.

- Food: Your brain needs stable blood sugar and essential nutrients to function well. Crashes in energy lead to cravings and impulsive behaviour.

- Hydration & Exercise: Both support brain function and mental clarity.

When your body is well-rested, well-fed, and moving, your brain has the fuel it needs to stay strong under pressure.

**Building Brain-Friendly Habits**

To build better self-control, you don't need to be perfect - just strategic. Here are some simple brain-based approaches:

**1. Reduce friction for good habits.**

- Keep a book on your bed to encourage reading.
- Lay your clothes out the night before to promote exercise.
- Your brain loves ease - use it to your advantage.

**2. Increase friction for bad habits.**

- Delete distracting apps.
- Hide junk food.
- Turn off notifications.

Make the wrong choice just a little harder, and your brain will thank you.

**3. Practice "The Pause."**

Before acting on impulse, take 3 deep breaths. Ask: "Is this what I really want?"

Even a few seconds of space can shift your decision from emotional to intentional.

### 4. Reward the right behaviors.

Celebrate small wins. Track your progress. Your brain responds well to **encouragement**.

### The Mind You Train is the Mind You Live With

Self-control is not a gift. It's a skill you develop by training your brain, managing your body, and building the right systems.

The more you practice conscious choices, the more your brain adapts. You'll find that temptations weaken, focus sharpens, and peace becomes more natural.

In time, the things that once pulled you off-track will lose their power - not because you fought them harder, but because you've grown stronger inside.

---

### Final Thoughts

The science of self-control teaches us a simple truth:

You are not just a passenger in your brain. You're the driver.

By understanding how your brain works - how dopamine, habits, stress, and decision-making intertwine - you gain the ability to reshape your life from the inside out.

In the next chapter, we'll explore a powerful paradox: how discipline, something most people resist, can actually create a life of greater freedom and joy. Because when you control your mind, you control your world.

# Chapter 4

# Freedom Through Discipline – A Paradox That Works

The idea of **discipline** often feels uncomfortable, reminding us of rigid schedules, rules, and restrictions. To many, it sounds like the opposite of **freedom**.

But here's one of life's most powerful paradoxes:

**True freedom is only possible through discipline.**

In this chapter, we'll explore why discipline isn't your enemy - it's your greatest ally. It's not about being strict for the sake of it. It's about building a strong inner foundation that gives you more energy, peace, clarity, and ultimately, more freedom than ever before.

### The Illusion of Freedom

We live in a world that glorifies personal freedom - the ability to do whatever we want, whenever we want. But without discipline, this kind of freedom becomes chaos.

Here's what often happens:

- You stay up late scrolling social media.
- You eat whatever feels good in the moment.
- You avoid hard tasks because they're uncomfortable.

In the short term, this feels like freedom. No one's telling you what to do. But over time, it leads to:

- Fatigue and poor sleep.
- Health issues or low energy.
- Guilt, regret, and unfinished goals.

This is not freedom. It's slavery to impulse.

**The Truth About Discipline**

Let's redefine discipline, not as punishment, but as preparation.

Discipline is the daily practice of choosing what you want most over what you want now.

It's the quiet commitment to your values. It's the structure you create so you can do what matters without being constantly pulled by emotion or distraction.

Discipline gives you:

- Freedom from guilt – because you know you've done your best.
- Freedom from chaos – because your time is intentional.
- Freedom to grow – because you're not stuck in cycles of regret.

## Discipline Builds Confidence

One of the most beautiful things about self-discipline is that it builds self-trust.

Every time you follow through on a promise to yourself - whether it's waking up on time, exercising, or avoiding that second helping - you prove to yourself that you are in control.

And that quiet inner voice says:

"If I can do this, I can do more."

That's how confidence is born - not from motivational speeches, but from small, daily acts of discipline.

## The Real-Life Power of Structure

Structure is the external reflection of discipline. It's how you set up your environment, routines, and priorities to support your goals - rather than sabotage them.

Let's look at a few examples:

1. Morning Routines

A solid morning routine is a disciplined way to start your day on your terms. It removes decision fatigue and creates momentum.

Even something simple like:

- Wake up at a fixed time
- Meditate or journal for 5 minutes
- Stretch or drink water

... can train your brain to enter the day with intention and calm.

2. Digital Boundaries

Your devices are tools - but without discipline, they dominate your attention. Creating screen-free times, using app blockers, or setting phone-free hours restores your mental space and focus.

3. Intentional Planning

Discipline isn't just about avoiding bad habits. It's about scheduling the right ones. Planning your week with even a loose structure allows your time to reflect your values, not just your moods.

**The Athlete's Secret**

Top performers in any field - athletes, artists, and entrepreneurs, all understand one truth:

**Discipline = Freedom to perform at your best.**

An athlete doesn't train every day because they enjoy pain. They train because they want to be free on game day - free to play at their highest potential without fear or doubt.

The same principle applies to life:

- The disciplined writer is free to express without blocks.
- The disciplined musician is free to improvise without hesitation.

- The disciplined student is free to recall knowledge under pressure.

## Discipline Feels Hard... At First

Building discipline is uncomfortable in the beginning.

### Why is it hard?

Your brain is wired for comfort and ease. It prefers familiar patterns - even if they're harmful - over unfamiliar growth.

Just like muscles grow with resistance, mental strength grows with each disciplined choice. Eventually, what once felt hard becomes your new normal.

Examples of Discipline Becoming Natural

- Sleeping early becomes natural.
- Saying "no" becomes empowering.
- Prioritizing your goals becomes exciting.

Discipline becomes freedom on autopilot.

## A Simple Analogy: The Riverbanks

Imagine a powerful river with no banks. It floods, spills everywhere, and causes destruction.

Now picture that same river with solid banks - its flow becomes **focused, useful**, and **powerful**. It irrigates fields, generates electricity, and supports life.

That's what discipline does to your energy, time, and attention. It channels it, gives it direction, and transforms your potential into power.

## Final Thoughts

Discipline is not about living a restricted life. It's about creating a life where you feel strong, clear, and in control.

It may seem paradoxical, but it's true:

The more disciplined you become, the more freedom you feel.

### Types of Freedom Gained Through Discipline

- Freedom to say no to what doesn't serve you.
- Freedom to pursue your dreams without distraction.
- Freedom to live with peace, purpose, and presence.

As you move into the next part of the book - **Mastering Mind & Emotions** - you'll learn how discipline becomes even more powerful when combined with emotional intelligence, thought awareness, and the ability to delay gratification.

Your future is waiting, and discipline is the key that unlocks the door.

# PART -2

## Mastering Mind & Emotions

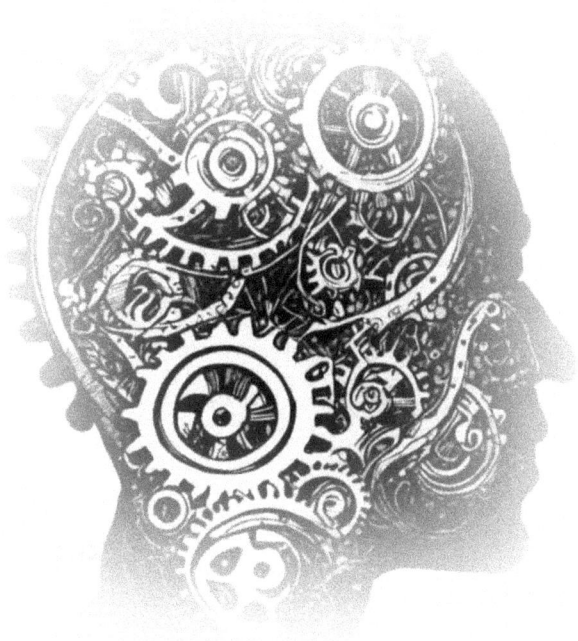

# Chapter 5

# Emotional Intelligence – The Secret to Inner Peace

If you've ever regretted saying something in anger, felt overwhelmed by stress, or struggled to stay calm during conflict, you already know this truth:

**Mastering your emotions is essential** to mastering yourself.

Self-control isn't just about resisting temptations or building routines - it's about managing what's going on *inside you*. And that's where **emotional intelligence** (EQ) comes in.

While IQ might measure your ability to solve problems, EQ determines how well you navigate life - your relationships, your inner peace, your decision-making. In this chapter, we'll explore how developing emotional intelligence becomes the bridge between self-control and lasting happiness.

### What Is Emotional Intelligence?

Emotional Intelligence is your ability to:

- **Recognize** your own emotions
- **Understand** what they're telling you
- **Manage** your reactions in healthy ways
- **Perceive and respond** to others' emotions with empathy

It's like having an *internal compass* - guiding you to stay calm under pressure, communicate clearly, and handle life's ups and downs without falling apart.

And here's the best part: just like self-discipline, **emotional intelligence can be developed**.

## Why Emotions Can Hijack Self-Control

Think of emotions like signals - they're data, not directions. But many people treat emotions as *orders*:

- Feel angry? Lash out.
- Feel sad? Withdraw.
- Feel anxious? Avoid the task.

Without emotional intelligence, your feelings become the **driver**, and your goals take the back seat.

The truth is, emotions are meant to be *noticed* - not *obeyed blindly*. That's the difference between **reacting** and **responding**. Self-control gives you the space to choose the latter.

## The 4 Pillars of Emotional Intelligence

Let's break EQ into four practical components that you can strengthen daily:

### 1. Self-Awareness

Recognizing your emotions as they arise.
Ask yourself: *"What am I feeling right now?"* or *"Why am I reacting this way?"*

Building this awareness turns unconscious habits into conscious choices. You can't control what you don't see.

**Practice Tip:** Pause throughout the day to name your emotions without judgment. Use phrases like: "I'm noticing irritation" instead of "I'm angry." This creates distance and clarity.

## 2. Self-Management

Once you're aware of your feelings, the next step is managing your reactions. This doesn't mean suppressing emotions - it means expressing them constructively.

Examples:

- Taking a walk when frustrated instead of snapping at someone
- Breathing deeply before replying to criticism
- Channeling sadness into journaling or creative work

**Key Insight:**
Self-control isn't denying your feelings - it's directing them.

## 3. Social Awareness

This is your ability to understand what others are feeling - through body language, tone, or energy - even if they don't say it.

Why this matters:
Understanding others' emotional states helps you respond with *empathy instead of ego*.

**Practice Tip:** When in conversation, shift your focus from "What should I say next?" to "What is this person really feeling?"
Listening is a superpower.

## 4. Relationship Management

**EQ in action** means handling conflict with grace, giving feedback without harm, and inspiring others through calm leadership.

Whether it's your partner, coworker, or friend - your ability to remain steady in emotional moments deepens trust and connection.

**Remember:** Relationships thrive not when you're always "right," but when you're consistently centered.

## The Inner Peace Equation

Let's bring it all together:

**Self-awareness + self-regulation = inner peace.**

When you're no longer controlled by mood swings, emotional triggers, or other people's energy, something magical happens:

You feel stable. Grounded. Calm even during storms.

And that's not just a nice feeling - it's a massive source of freedom. Because now, your peace is no longer at the mercy of the outside world.

**How to Train Emotional Intelligence**

Just like you train muscles, you can train emotional intelligence with consistent small practices. Here are a few:

1. **The Name-It Game**: When you feel overwhelmed, name what you're feeling. Use specific labels like: "disappointed," "embarrassed," "insecure." Naming the emotion reduces its grip.

2. **The 90-Second Rule**: According to neuroscientist Dr. Jill Bolte Taylor, when you have an emotional reaction, it physically lasts about 90 seconds. If you don't feed it with thoughts, it will pass on its own. So, the next time you feel triggered, wait 90 seconds. Breathe. Let the wave roll through. Then choose your response.

3. **The Emotion Journal**: At the end of each day, write:

- What strong emotions did I feel today?
- What triggered them?
- How did I respond?
- What could I do differently next time?

This builds self-awareness like nothing else.

## Emotional Intelligence & Self-Control

When your emotional intelligence is strong:

- You don't say things that you'll regret later.
- You don't sabotage progress because of temporary moods.
- You don't overreact or freeze up in chaos.

Instead, you stay in control - not by suppressing emotions, but by understanding and channeling them. This is the secret to real power: calm in the midst of pressure, clarity in the middle of noise.

---

## Final Thoughts

**Emotional intelligence** isn't weakness, it's **strategic strength**.

It helps you build stronger relationships, make wiser decisions, and create a stable inner world that doesn't collapse at the first sign of stress.

When you manage your emotions, you manage your life.

And from that foundation, happiness becomes not just possible - it becomes sustainable.

In the next chapter, we'll explore a superpower that emotional intelligence makes easier:

**The Art of Delayed Gratification** - where patience becomes a pathway to long-term joy.

# Chapter 6

# The Art of Delayed Gratification – Patience Pays Off

**What would you choose?** If offered a choice between Rs.100 right now or Rs. 1000 a month from now, most people say, "Rs. 1000, of course." However, in real-life situations, they often choose the immediate reward. Why?

Because **delayed gratification** is easy to understand but hard to practice. It's a powerful tool for self-control and a cornerstone of lasting happiness.

In this chapter, we'll explore how delaying short-term pleasure leads to long-term joy and how you can train yourself to become a master of patience in an impatient world.

**The Marshmallow Test**

In the 1970s, a famous psychological experiment known as the Marshmallow Test was conducted. Children were given one marshmallow and told they could eat it immediately or wait 15 minutes to receive two marshmallows.

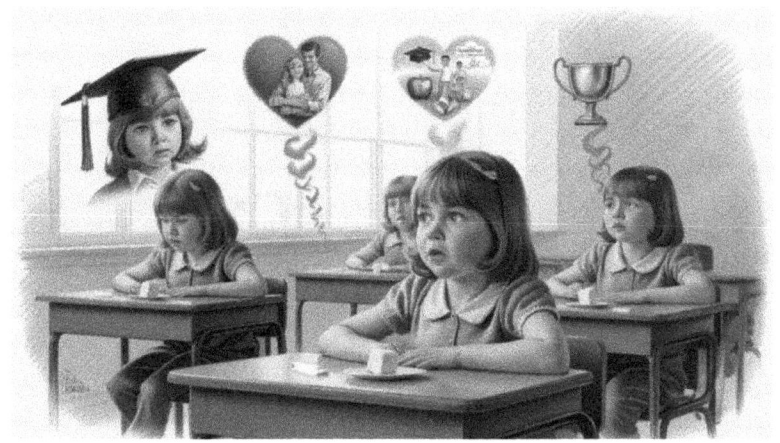

The results?

**Those who waited had:**

- Higher academic performance
- Better health
- More fulfilling relationships
- Greater career success

The key difference wasn't intelligence or background; it was **self-control** - the ability to wait and say "no" now for a bigger "yes" later.

**Why the Brain Craves Instant Rewards**

Your brain has two key systems at play:

1. The **Limbic System** (emotional brain) – seeks pleasure, avoids pain, acts now.
2. The **Prefrontal Cortex** (rational brain) – plans ahead, weighs consequences, thinks long-term.

When you delay gratification, you strengthen your prefrontal cortex - responsible for decision-making, self-discipline, and goal setting.

It's like this:

Every time you choose long-term gain over short-term pleasure; your brain rewires itself for success.

**Examples in Daily Life**

Here are real-world situations where delaying gratification pays off:

- Health: Skipping sugary snacks today → long-term energy, fitness, and vitality.
- Finance: Saving money instead of impulsive spending → freedom from debt and future security.
- Career: Focusing on deep work now → mastery, promotions, and fulfillment later.
- Relationships: Holding back harsh words → deeper connection and mutual respect over time.

The formula is simple:

- Short-term pain = long-term gain

- Short-term pleasure = long-term regret

## The Hidden Joy of Waiting

Delayed gratification isn't just about sacrifice - it's about savoring.

Think about it:

- The vacation you planned and saved for? Feels richer.
- The dessert after a week of clean eating? Tastes better.
- The reward after a long struggle? Feels earned.

Waiting intensifies appreciation. Patience deepens pleasure.

When you stop grabbing every quick fix, you make space for deeper joy - the kind that doesn't vanish as soon as the moment passes.

## Training Yourself to Delay Gratification

This is a skill - and like all skills, it grows with practice. Here are a few ways to build it:

### 1. Micro-Delays

Start small.

- Wait 10 minutes before eating that snack.
- Delay replying to that angry message for 5 minutes.
- Sit in silence for 2 minutes before starting your day.

Each small pause strengthens your discipline muscle.

## 2. Visualize the Long-Term Reward

Remind yourself why you're saying no to the now.

Whether it's a healthier body, financial freedom, or peace of mind - keep the future benefit vivid in your mind.

Write it down. Create a vision board. Make it real.

## 3. Remove the Temptation

**Don't rely on willpower alone.** Design your environment for success.

Consider these strategies:

- Avoid keeping junk food at home if you're trying to eat clean.
- Block distracting apps when working.
- Keep your savings out of easy access.

**Out of sight = out of mind = easier self-control.**

## 4. Reward Yourself - Strategically

Delayed gratification doesn't mean denying pleasure forever.

It means earn it, enjoy it, and move on.

Set milestones and reward yourself mindfully. This keeps motivation alive.

## Delayed Gratification in Spiritual Traditions

Ancient philosophies and spiritual teachings have long promoted restraint, fasting, simplicity, and detachment. Why?

Because they understood a timeless truth:

Inner peace comes not from indulging every desire, but from mastering them.

Whether it's the Buddha under the Bodhi tree, or monks in silent meditation, the message is the same:

Real joy is found not in reacting to every urge - but in transcending them.

## The Happiness Link

Here's the connection between **delayed gratification** and ultimate happiness:

When you train yourself to wait - to pause, to reflect, to act with purpose - you:

- Build **inner strength**
- Gain **long-term rewards**
- Feel **proud** of your choices
- Avoid **regret**

- Trust **yourself** more
- Live with **intention**

This is a different kind of happiness - not the rush of dopamine, but the quiet joy of knowing you're becoming who you want to be.

---

## Final Thoughts

In a world of "same-day delivery," "one-click purchase," and instant everything, **patience feels radical**. But it's also liberating.

The ability to **delay gratification** is the ability to create your future.

With every patient choice, you're not just resisting - you're investing, in your **health**, your **peace**, your **dreams**.

And one day, when the rewards show up - you'll realize: it was worth every moment of the wait.

# Chapter 7

# Breaking Addictions – Escaping the Instant Gratification Trap

We live in the age of addiction.

Not just to substances - but to **screens, snacks, likes, online shopping, gossip, constant noise, and instant approval**. Anything that gives a quick hit of pleasure can become a trap.

If you've ever said "just five minutes" and lost an hour scrolling, or found yourself reaching for junk food even when you're not hungry - you've tasted the pull of instant gratification.

But here's the truth:

Addiction isn't about the thing itself. It's about your *relationship* with it.

And once you understand how addiction hijacks your brain and emotions, you can take your power back - step by step.

This chapter is about breaking free from those invisible chains and reclaiming control over your choices, your focus, and your future.

## What Is Addiction, really?

Addiction isn't just chemical dependency. At its core, addiction is:

- Compulsive **behavior**
- That brings **short-term relief**
- But it creates **long-term harm**

You know it's not helping - yet you keep returning. Why?

Because it becomes your escape from stress, boredom, pain, or emptiness. But instead of solving the problem, it **amplifies it** and then traps you in a loop.

## The Brain's Reward System

Every time you engage in a pleasurable activity, your brain releases **dopamine** - the "feel-good" chemical.

The problem? Highly stimulating activities like junk food, video games, social media, or binge-watching release unnatural amounts of dopamine - much more than healthy behaviors like walking, reading, or connecting with someone face-to-face.

Over time, your brain:

- Gets used to high dopamine levels
- Craves more stimulation to feel normal
- Find regular activities dull or boring

This is how instant gratification becomes **enslavement**. You don't feel joy - you feel **numb** unless you're chasing that next hit.

**Common Modern Addictions (Beyond Substances)**

You may not be hooked on alcohol or cigarettes, but ask yourself:

- Do I check my phone compulsively, even when I don't need to?
- Do I eat or shop when I feel sad, stressed, or bored?
- Do I struggle to spend even 10 minutes in silence?

If yes - you're not alone. The modern world is designed to keep you addicted - to convenience, consumption, comparison, and control.

But here's the good news:

Awareness is the first step to freedom.

**The Real Cost of Addiction**

Addictions may bring momentary comfort, but they:

- Weaken self-control
- Distract you from your goals
- Drain time, energy, and money
- Widen the gap between who you are and who you want to be

They create a life where you're always reacting – not choosing.
Surviving - not thriving.

## Escaping the Trap: 6 Powerful Steps

### 1. Acknowledge the Addiction Without Shame

Don't fight it with guilt or denial. That only strengthens the cycle.

Instead, say: "I'm caught in a habit that doesn't serve me anymore. I want something better."

Compassion unlocks change faster than self-criticism.

### 2. Understand Your Triggers

Every addiction has a cue - a moment that sparks the craving.

It could be:

- Emotional (stress, loneliness, boredom)
- Situational (late nights, scrolling before bed)
- Environmental (certain places, smells, or sounds)

Track what leads you into the loop. Awareness creates distance.

### 3. Replace, Don't Just Remove

You can't just stop a habit - you need to replace it with a healthier alternative.

Examples:

- Craving junk food → Drink a glass of water and eat fruit
- Mindless scrolling → Read 2 pages of a book or stretch
- Feeling anxious → Practice 2 minutes of deep breathing

Your brain still wants relief. Give it something nourishing.

## 4. Delay the Urge

Use the **5-Minute Rule**: When an urge hits, wait 5 minutes before acting on it. During that time, do something else - walk, breathe, journal.

More often than not, the urge will pass. You just need to outlast the wave.

## 5. Create Friction

Make it harder to engage with the addictive habit:

- Log out of apps
- Delete shortcuts
- Use grayscale mode on your phone
- Don't keep snacks in easy reach

When a habit is harder to access, you're less likely to fall into it.

## 6. Celebrate Progress, Not Perfection

You don't have to be flawless. You just need to be **more in control today than yesterday**.

Even if you slip, reflect - don't punish. What did you learn? What can you do differently next time?

Each small victory strengthens your identity as someone who is **free**.

## The Deepest Need Behind Every Addiction

Here's a powerful truth:

Behind every addictive behavior is a legitimate emotional need.

You don't need more control - you need more connection, purpose, rest, love, and peace.

The question isn't: "How do I stop?" It's: *"What am I really craving?"*

The more you meet your true needs - the less power the false highs will have over you.

## Breaking Free = Reclaiming Joy

When you reduce your reliance on instant pleasure, something beautiful happens:

- You start to enjoy the little things again
- You feel more present
- You regain your energy, time, and self-respect

You no longer feel like life is dragging you around.
**You are back in the driver's seat.**

And that, in itself, is happiness.

---

**Final Thoughts**

You don't have to be perfect to be free. You just have to **decide that your future is more important than your impulses.**

Every time you choose presence over distraction, nourishment over indulgence, growth over comfort - you heal.

And with each healed part of yourself, your ability to experience **deep, lasting happiness** grows stronger.

Freedom is not the absence of desire. It's the ability to choose *what* to desire - and when.

In the next chapter, we'll explore how to train your thoughts - the silent shapers of your emotions, actions, and habits.

# Chapter 8

# Training Your Thoughts – From Chaos to Clarity

*"What you consistently think shapes what you say;*
*What you say guides what you do;*
*What you do forms your habits;*
*And your habits shape the course of your life."*

Our lives are shaped by what we repeatedly think. Yet most of us are never taught how to think. We're flooded with opinions, media, fears, and past conditioning - and without awareness, our minds become noisy, reactive, and overwhelmed.

But here's the powerful truth:

You don't have to believe every thought you think. You can train your mind - just like your body.

This chapter is about turning your mind from a battlefield into a garden - a place where clarity, calm, and purpose grow.

**The Nature of Thought**

The average person has **60,000–80,000 thoughts per day**. Most are:

- Repetitive
- Negative

- Unconscious

We worry about the future, replay the past, judge ourselves, compare with others. We get caught in loops like:

- "I'm not good enough."
- "What if I fail?"
- "They're better than me."
- "I'll never change."

These thoughts may feel *real*, but they aren't always *true*.

Thoughts are not facts - they are habits.

The good news? Habits can be changed.


## Why Mental Clarity Is Essential for Self-Control

Imagine trying to steer a boat in a storm - waves crashing, wind blowing, no compass. That's what it feels like trying to live intentionally without clarity of thought.

Mental chaos leads to:

- Emotional instability
- Poor decision-making
- Stress and anxiety
- Lack of focus and discipline

On the other hand, a trained mind is like calm water - you can see clearly, act wisely, and stay steady no matter what's happening outside.

## Step 1: Become the Watcher of Your Thoughts

The first step is to notice your thoughts - without judgment.

You are *not* your thoughts. You are the awareness behind them.

Start by observing:

- What thoughts arise when you wake up?
- What beliefs run through your head during stress?
- What stories do you tell yourself about success, failure, love, or your worth?

Awareness creates distance. Distance creates choice.

## Step 2: Challenge & Replace Negative Thinking

Once you catch a recurring thought, ask:

1. Is this thought true?
2. Is it helpful?
3. What's a better thought I can choose instead?

Examples:

- "I always mess things up." Relace with "I've made mistakes, but I'm learning and growing."
- "I'm too lazy." Relace with "I can take small steps and build momentum."
- "Nothing will ever change." Relace with "Every day is a fresh opportunity."

You're not lying to yourself - you're choosing thoughts that *empower* rather than *paralyze*.

**Step 3: Feed Your Mind with Better Input**

You can't plant roses in a garden full of weeds.

Protect your mind by choosing:

- Books that uplift and challenge you
- People who inspire rather than drain
- Media that educates, not agitates
- Self-talk that is kind and constructive

What you consume mentally is as important as what you eat physically.

**Step 4: Use Affirmations with Emotion**

Affirmations aren't magic spells - they're mental reps.

Pick 2–3 statements that reflect who you want to become. For example:

- "I am calm, focused, and in control."
- "I choose progress over perfection."
- "I trust myself to make wise decisions."

Say them aloud, feel them, visualize them. The more emotional energy you put in, the faster your mind accepts the new reality.

## Step 5: Practice Thought Stopping

When your mind starts spiraling into anxiety, comparison, or negativity - use a pattern interrupt.

Say to yourself:

- "Pause."
- "Not helpful."
- "Switch."

Then redirect to something constructive - gratitude, breath, or action.

You're not suppressing thoughts - you're refusing to fuel ones that lead nowhere.

## Step 6: Journal Your Mind Daily

Journaling is a powerful way to clear mental clutter.

Each morning or night, write:

- What am I thinking about?
- What's stressing me?
- What do I want to focus on instead?

Even 5 minutes of stream-of-consciousness writing can create mental spaciousness - making it easier to reflect instead of react.

## Step 7: Meditate for Mental Discipline

Meditation is not about "emptying your mind." It's about **training attention**.

Start with 5–10 minutes a day:

- Sit quietly.
- Focus on your breath.
- When thoughts come, gently bring attention back.

This builds the skill of **awareness + redirection** - the foundation of self-control.

Over time, meditation rewires your brain for:

- Calm
- Focus
- Emotional regulation
- Greater inner clarity

**Thoughts Shape Emotions, Emotions Shape Actions**

Every emotion starts as a thought. Every action starts as a feeling.

When you train your thoughts:

- You regulate your moods
- You make better decisions
- You stay focused on what truly matters

It's not about becoming a robot. It's about being conscious, not controlled.

**Final Thoughts**

A chaotic mind creates a chaotic life. A trained mind creates a life of meaning, peace, and power.

You can't always control what thoughts come in. But you can choose which ones stay.

By cultivating a daily practice of awareness, reflection, and redirection, you move from mental noise to mental mastery - from reaction to intention.

This is the inner foundation of lasting happiness.

In the next part of the book, we'll take these inner principles and apply them to daily life - where habits, routines, and real-world choices shape our destiny.

# PART -3

## Self-Control in Daily Life

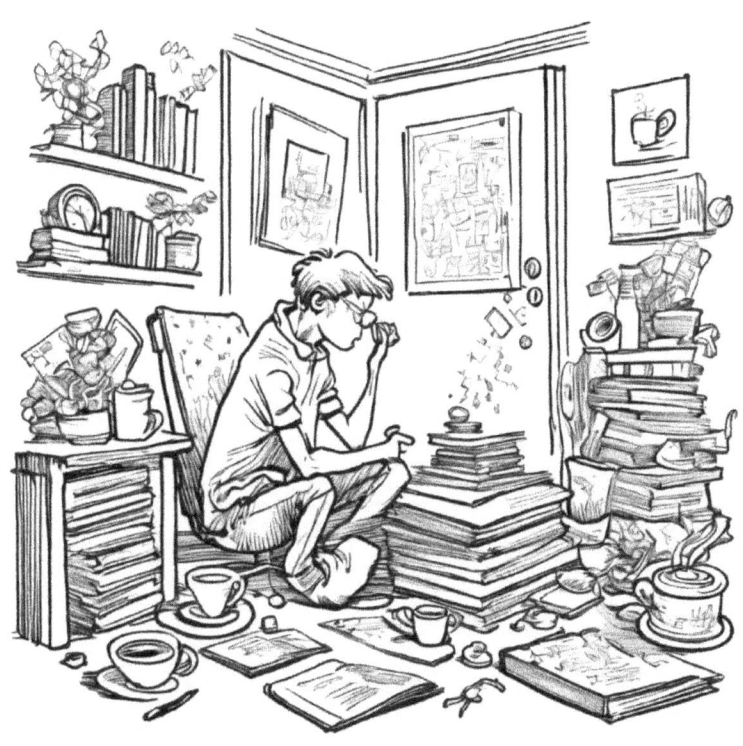

# Chapter 9

# Mastering Habits –

# Small Changes, Big Impact

*"It's not the future we choose directly, but the habits we build- and those habits are what ultimately shape our future."*

If your life is a movie, then **habits are the script**. They run quietly in the background, shaping how you think, feel, and act - without needing permission.

Whether it's brushing your teeth, reaching for your phone, procrastinating, exercising, or overthinking - it's all habit.

So, if self-control feels hard, it's not because you're weak. It's because your current habits are running on autopilot.

The secret?

**Small daily habits** are the invisible architecture of success, happiness, and freedom.

In this chapter, we'll learn how to build, break, and master habits - the foundation of real self-control.

## What Exactly Is a Habit?

A **habit** is a behavior that becomes automatic through repetition.
It follows a loop:

1. **Cue** – a trigger (time, emotion, place)
2. **Craving** – your desire or urge
3. **Response** – the action you take
4. **Reward** – the benefit you get (pleasure, relief, comfort)

This loop runs silently all day long. The more you repeat it, the stronger it becomes.

To change your life, you don't need to change everything. You just need to **shift the loop**.


## Why Habits Matter More Than Motivation

Motivation is **temporary** - it depends on your mood.

Habits are **reliable** - they work even when you're tired, lazy, or uninspired.

That's why the most successful people don't rely on willpower. They build systems that run their lives for them.

Discipline becomes effortless when you design your environment and identity around the habits you want.

## Step 1: Start Tiny

One of the biggest mistakes people make is trying to change everything at once.

Instead, ask: **"What's the smallest version of this habit I can start with?"**

- Want to meditate? Start with **1 minute**
- Want to exercise? Do **1 push-up**
- Want to write a journal? Write **one sentence**

Tiny wins build confidence. Consistency builds momentum.

Small changes are sustainable. Big changes are emotional and often short-lived.

**Step 2: Stack Your Habits**

Want to build a new habit? Attach it to one that already exists. This is called **habit stacking**.

Formula: **After I [current habit], I will [new habit].**

Examples:

- After I brush my teeth → I'll say 1 positive affirmation
- After I eat lunch → I'll Walk for 5 minutes
- After I shut my laptop → I'll spend 2 minutes in silence

This creates a natural flow - and makes the new habit easier to remember and do.

**Step 3: Make It Obvious, Easy, and Rewarding**

Design your environment to support your new habit:

- Keep your book next to your pillow
- Put your yoga mat where you'll see it
- Lay out workout clothes the night before

- Delete distracting apps from your home screen

And when you complete the habit - **celebrate**! Smile, fist pump, say "yes!" aloud.

Your brain loves rewards. Even small ones reinforce the behavior.

### Step 4: Don't Break the Chain

Make it a game:

**"How many days in a row can I do this?"**

Use a wall calendar, habit tracker app, or notebook. Each day you complete your habit, **mark an X**.

You'll find yourself doing it just to keep the streak alive. That's how habit becomes identity. If you miss a day - no problem. Just never miss *two* in a row. That's the danger zone.

### Step 5: Watch the Language of Identity

The strongest habits are built on identity. Not "I want to..." But: **"I am the kind of person who..."**

- Not: "I want to eat healthy"
- Instead: "I am someone who takes care of my body"
- Not: "I'll try to read more"
- Instead: "I am a reader"

When you change your identity, your habits follow. And every small win reinforces the new identity.

## Step 6: Break Bad Habits with Inversion

To break a habit, **invert the loop**:

1. **Make the cue invisible**

    – Out of sight = out of mind

    – Example: Keep snacks off your desk, turn off app notifications

2. **Make the craving unattractive**

    – Reframe: "This isn't relaxing, it's numbing"

    – Highlight long-term pain over short-term pleasure

3. **Make the response difficult**

    – Add friction: Log out, use screen timers, block websites

    – The harder it is, the less likely it happens

4. **Make the reward unsatisfying**

    – Track the cost: money wasted, time lost, energy drained

    – Create accountability with a friend or group

## Compounding Power: The 1% Rule

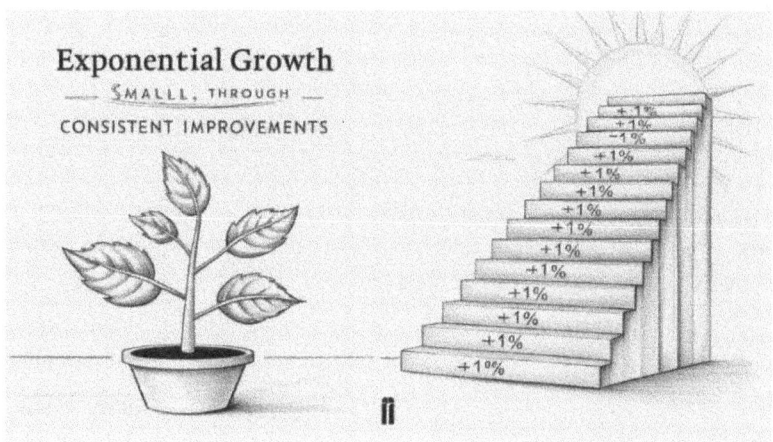

Improving by just 1% every day doesn't seem like much. But over a year? **You become 37 times better.**

That's the magic of compounding. Small changes, consistently applied, create massive transformation over time.

Success is rarely the result of big breakthroughs. It's the result of tiny smart choices repeated daily.

---

## Final Thoughts

Self-control isn't about being rigid or perfect. It's about making daily decisions that reflect who you truly want to be.

And it all starts with habits - those invisible forces that either lift you or limit you.

You don't need a dramatic change. You need a small start - done consistently.

The habits you master today become the **freedom, focus, and happiness** you enjoy tomorrow.

In the next chapter, we'll take this idea further and explore how **routine** can turn discipline into a peaceful, powerful lifestyle.

# Chapter 10

# The Power of Routine – Turning Discipline into a Lifestyle

*"Success isn't just about aiming high with goals- it's about the systems you rely on, because when pressure hits, you lean on what you've built."*

If habits are individual building blocks, **routine is the structure they form** - your daily rhythm of life.

While habits are automatic, routines are intentional. They're a collection of habits woven together with purpose and flow.

A powerful routine doesn't restrict your freedom - it creates it. It frees your mind from constant decision-making and gives your energy to what really matters.

Routine is how self-control becomes second nature. It's how discipline turns into a lifestyle.

Let's explore how to design a daily life that supports clarity, peace, and purpose.

## Why Routine Works Like Magic

Our brain loves patterns. When we repeat a sequence regularly, our mind no longer has to think. This conserves energy and reduces stress.

Without routines, we suffer from:

- Decision fatigue: too many small choices sap willpower
- Scattered focus: constantly switching tasks
- Inconsistency: starting strong, then dropping off

With a strong routine, we gain:

- Mental clarity
- Emotional balance
- Physical rhythm
- Predictable results

In short - you stop living reactively and start living **intentionally**.

## Morning Routine: Win the First Hour

How you start your day sets the tone for everything else.

A mindful morning routine:

- Grounds your emotions
- Primes your focus
- Builds momentum

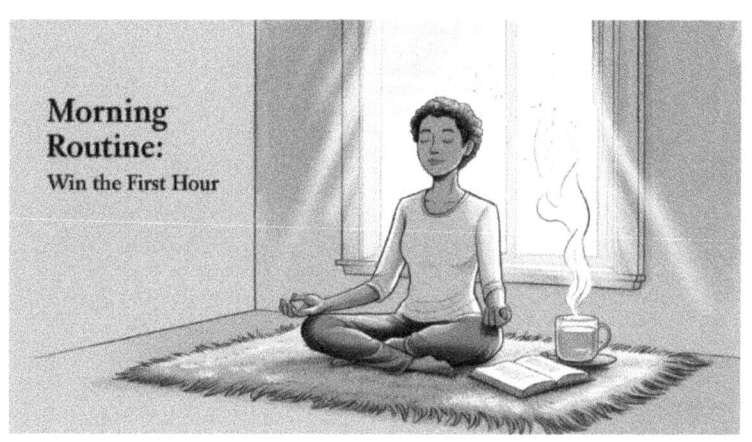

**Sample Morning Routine (30–60 mins):**

Even if you start with just 15 minutes, consistency is what matters.

1. Wake Up Early: Before the world demands your attention
2. Hydrate: Energize your body
3. Silence or Meditation: Calm your mind
4. Movement: Wake up your body (yoga, walk, stretches)
5. Journal or Reflect: Organize thoughts
6. Read or Learn: Feed your mind with wisdom
7. Set Intentions: Choose your focus for the day

**Evening Routine: Prepare for Peace**

Your evening routine is not just about winding down. It's about setting up tomorrow's success.

**Sample Evening Routine:**

A strong evening routine helps you sleep better and wake up with intention.

1. Digital Sunset: Turn off screens 30–60 mins before bed
2. Review Your Day: Reflect on wins & lessons
3. Plan Tomorrow: Decide on the top 3 priorities
4. Gratitude Practice: Write 3 things you're thankful for
5. Relaxation Ritual: Light reading, calming music, or breathing

**Anchoring Your Day with Micro-Routines**

Not every routine has to be long. Use **micro-routines** to regain focus throughout the day.

Examples:

- **Before a meeting** → 3 deep breaths
- **After lunch** → 5-min walk + water
- **Feeling stressed** → Quick journaling or pause

These tiny resets help you stay grounded and in control, especially during chaos.

**How to Build a Routine That Sticks**

Here's how to make your routine *yours*:

1. **Start simple**

    – Don't copy someone else's perfect day. Start with 2–3 anchor habits.

2. **Tie it to existing triggers**

    – "After I brush my teeth, I'll stretch."

    – "After I drink coffee, I'll plan my top 3 tasks."

3. **Prepare your environment**

    – Lay out clothes, prep your journal, cue the playlist - make it easy.

4. **Track and adjust**

    – Use a habit tracker, calendar, or simple checklist. Adapt what works.

5. **Make it enjoyable**

    – Add music, candles, nature, or anything that makes the process rewarding.

Discipline doesn't have to feel heavy. With the right flow, it becomes something you *look forward to*.

**What to Do When You Fall Off**

Life happens. Routines break. That's normal.

The trick is not to feel guilty, but to reset quickly.

Ask yourself:

- "What's the smallest version of my routine I can do today?"
- "How can I re-anchor myself with one micro habit?"

The goal isn't perfection - it's returning to alignment faster each time.

## Real-Life Examples of Routine Power

A writer who writes 500 words every morning, no matter what.
An athlete who stretches and visualizes before every practice.
A parent who spends 10 minutes reading to their child nightly.
A leader who starts the day with silence and journaling.

These routines aren't glamorous - but over time, they create mastery, peace, and meaningful results.

Success is never about one big moment. It's about what you repeat when no one's watching.

---

## Final Thoughts

Self-control isn't something you "turn on" when needed. It's something you **live through daily structure**.

A solid routine is the soil where discipline grows. It turns self-control from a force of effort into a **state of being**.

By designing your day with intention, you free your mind, protect your energy, and align your life with what truly matters.

In the next chapter, we'll explore how self-control strengthens our most important bonds - our relationships.

# Chapter 11

# Self-Control in Relationships – The Key to Deeper Connections

*"Every trigger gives us a moment-however brief-to choose our reaction. Within that moment lies our strength to grow, and the freedom to shape who we become."*

We often think of self-control as a personal discipline - something private, about our habits and inner battles.

But the truth is:

**Your relationships are the mirror of your self-control.**

Every interaction - with your partner, family, friends, colleagues - is an opportunity to either react or respond. To either inflame or heal. To either demand or understand.

And the quality of those choices? They define the depth, peace, and strength of your connections.

**Emotional Triggers & the Pause Button**

Everyone has emotional triggers: A rude comment, a late reply, a raised voice, a cold shoulder.

Without self-control, these triggers light up **automatic reactions** - snapping, blaming, withdrawing, or over-explaining.

But with self-awareness and discipline, we install a **pause button**.

That pause gives us space to:

- Feel the emotion without feeding it
- Respond rather than react
- Understand rather than assume
- Choose compassion over control

This pause is powerful. It creates safety in relationships. Safety leads to trust. Trust leads to depth.


**Listening: The Discipline of Presence**

One of the most overlooked self-control skills is **listening** - not just hearing, but truly being present.

When someone speaks, are you:

- Thinking of your reply?
- Waiting for your turn to talk?
- Judging silently?

Or are you fully *there*, listening without an agenda?

True listening is hard. It requires:

- Patience
- An open heart
- Control over your internal chatter

But it's also one of the most healing gifts you can offer someone.

People don't want to be fixed. They want to be seen, heard, and felt.

## Handling Conflict with Self-Control

Conflict is not a sign of failure. It's a sign of connection that needs refinement.

The problem isn't *if* we argue - but *how* we argue.

Without self-control:

- We blame and shame
- We escalate emotionally
- We bring up the past
- We withdraw or attack

With self-control:

- We focus on the issue, not the person
- We speak from feelings, not accusations
- We choose silence over sarcasm
- We aim to understand, not to win

When both people bring emotional maturity, conflict becomes a bridge - not a battlefield.

## Setting Boundaries: A Form of Self-Respect

Self-control in relationships also means knowing when to say *no* - without guilt.

You can't pour from an empty cup. If you're always pleasing others, suppressing your truth, or tolerating disrespect, you burn out.

Setting healthy boundaries takes courage and discipline. It might look like:

- Saying "I need space" instead of lashing out
- Choosing alone time instead of forced company
- Saying "no" to drama or gossip
- Not responding immediately to emotional demands

Boundaries are not walls. They're doors. They keep the wrong energy out and let the right ones in.


## The Power of Compassion & Forgiveness

When someone hurts you - intentionally or not - your natural reaction might be to strike back or withdraw.

But self-control allows you to pause, process, and choose the higher path.

Forgiveness is not weakness. It's the strength to say:

- "I choose peace over resentment."
- "I release you from my expectations."
- "I won't let this pain control me."

Forgiveness frees your heart and it makes space for authentic reconnection - with yourself and others.

## When to Speak, When to Stay Silent

Sometimes, saying nothing is an act of maturity. Other times, silence can be a form of avoidance.

Self-control helps you discern the difference.

**Speak when:**

- Your voice adds value, clarity, or truth
- Silence would build resentment
- You're calm enough to speak with love, not ego

**Stay silent when:**

- Emotions are too high to speak wisely
- You're tempted to defend rather than understand
- You're about to say something you'll regret

Words are like arrows. Once released, they can't be taken back. Master your words, and you master your relationships.

## Practicing Self-Control as Love

We often think love is about passion, attraction, or connection.

But love is also about **restraint**:

- Holding back a criticism

- Pausing before reacting
- Giving space instead of clinging
- Letting go instead of forcing

In this way, self-control becomes an act of love. It says:

"I care about our connection more than I care about being right."

"I'm choosing peace over pride."

"I'm creating a safe space for both of us to grow."

---

## Final Thoughts

Self-control isn't cold or robotic. In fact, it's the opposite - it's deeply human. It's about making conscious choices in the heat of emotion. It's about loving yourself and others enough to choose maturity over impulse.

Your relationships flourish not because you avoid problems, but because you bring presence, patience, and purpose to them.

And that is the true power of self-mastery.

In the next chapter, we'll look at how the same principle of control applies to our money and how financial discipline leads to peace, freedom, and success.

# Chapter 12

# Financial Self-Control – Wealth, Success & Peace of Mind

*"Don't treat saving as an afterthought—save first, and use what remains for spending."*

Money is a tool - a neutral one. It's not good or bad. It simply **amplifies your choices**.

But when left unchecked, money becomes a major source of stress, anxiety, and even relationship breakdowns and at the heart of most money problems?

A lack of self-control.

Whether it's impulsive spending, chasing status, or delaying important financial goals - it all comes back to discipline.

Financial self-control isn't about being cheap. It's about being **intentional**. It's about choosing long-term peace over short-term pleasure.

**The Impulse Trap: Why We Overspend**

Everywhere we go, we're bombarded with messages telling us:

- "You deserve it."

- "Buy now, pay later."
- "Treat yourself."

It's easy to confuse **wants** with **needs**, and **self-worth** with what we own.

Impulse spending gives a dopamine rush - a momentary high. But like any addiction, it often leaves behind:

- Regret
- Clutter
- Debt
- Anxiety

**Financial freedom** isn't about how much you earn - it's about how much you *keep* and how well you manage it.

**Step 1: Know Where Your Money Goes**

You can't control what you don't track. The first step toward financial discipline is simple:

**Awareness = Power**

Make a habit of tracking your monthly expenses. You don't need fancy apps - a basic notebook or spreadsheet works.

Divide your spending into categories:

- Essentials (food, rent, bills)
- Wants (eating out, shopping, gadgets)
- Savings & investments

- Debt repayments
- Giving (charity, support)

This will show you *exactly* where your money leaks - and where you can course-correct.

## Step 2: Build a Simple Budget

A budget is not a punishment. It's a **freedom plan**. It tells your money where to go, instead of wondering where it went.

Here's a basic rule: **50-30-20 Rule**

- 50% – Essentials
- 30% – Wants
- 20% – Savings/Investments

But you can adjust based on your lifestyle and goals. The key is to **prioritize savings and debt freedom**, not just consumption.

Budgeting builds mindfulness - every expense becomes a conscious decision.

## Step 3: Delay Gratification

Financial discipline is deeply connected to **delayed gratification**.

Ask yourself before a purchase:

- "Do I really need this?"

- "Will this still matter in a month?"
- "Am I buying this out of boredom or insecurity?"

Use the **24-Hour Rule**: If you want to buy something non-essential, wait a day. Most of the time, the urge will pass.

Over time, you shift from being a **consumer** to a **creator** of value.

## Step 4: Save Before You Spend

One of the best habits you can build: **Pay yourself first.**

As soon as you receive income:

- Set aside a fixed % for savings (start with 10–20%)
- Automate it if possible
- Treat it as a *non-negotiable bill*

This single habit creates a financial cushion - and peace of mind.

Even small savings done consistently build wealth over time.

## Step 5: Kill Debt, Slowly & Steadily

Debt creates mental clutter. It weighs down your present and robs your future.

Make a plan to eliminate it:

- List all your debts
- Start with the smallest or highest interest

- Pay extra toward one while maintaining the rest
- Celebrate each win

Freedom from debt isn't just financial - it's **emotional liberation**.

**Step 6: Invest in Your Future Self**

Spending can feel good now. But **investing** feels good long-term.

This doesn't just mean stocks or mutual funds (though those matter too).

It means:

- Learning new skills
- Attending workshops
- Starting a side hustle
- Building assets, not liabilities

Financial self-control means asking: "Will this purchase serve me today *and* tomorrow?"

Choose growth over gratification.

**Step 7: Redefine Wealth**

Wealth isn't just about a bank balance. It's about having:

- Time freedom
- Peace of mind

- The ability to help others
- A life free from financial anxiety

You're rich when your lifestyle matches your values - not your income.

You're rich when your joy isn't tied to what you buy. You're rich when your money habits reflect inner peace.

---

**Final Thoughts**

Financial self-control isn't about saying "no" forever - it's about saying "yes" to what truly matters.

It's choosing clarity over chaos, value over vanity, and freedom over fleeting pleasure.

Master your money - and you'll gain more than just wealth. You'll gain **confidence**, **security**, and the ability to live life on your terms.


In the final part of this book, we'll shift gears and explore the ultimate reward of self-control - not just success or discipline, but something deeper: **lasting happiness.**

# PART -4

## The Ultimate Reward –
## True Happiness

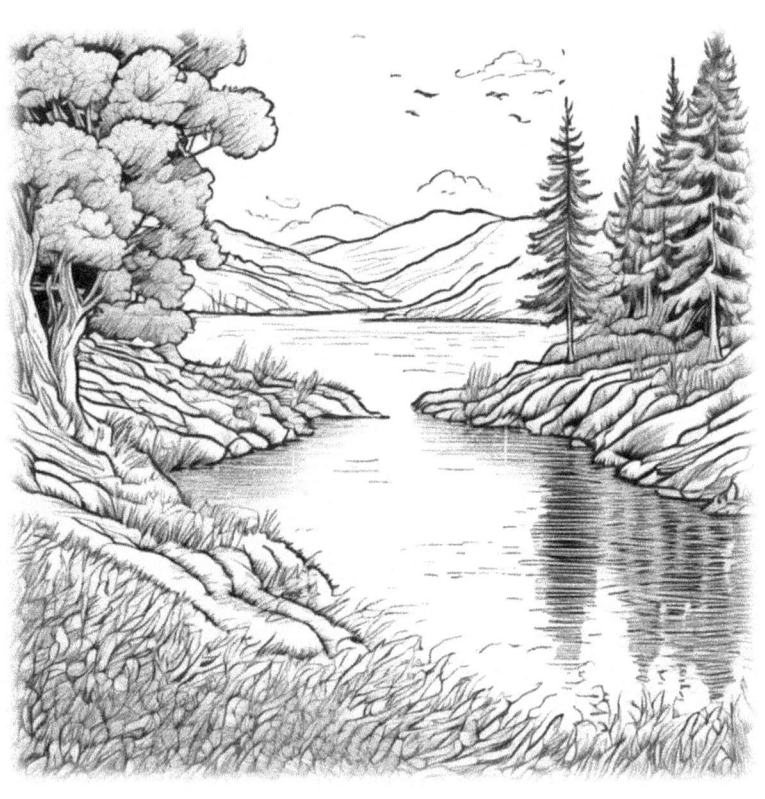

# Chapter 13

# The Joy of Saying No – Protecting Your Energy

For most of us, saying "no" feels uncomfortable. We're afraid of hurting others, missing out, or being seen as selfish.

So we say "yes" - to things we don't want, don't need, and don't believe in. Over time, this drains our energy, clouds our clarity, and leaves us feeling resentful and overwhelmed.

But here's the truth:

**Every 'yes' is a 'no' to something else** and often, that something is *you*.

Learning to say **no with grace** is one of the most powerful acts of self-control - and one of the greatest keys to true happiness.

**Why We Struggle to Say No**

We're trained from childhood to please others. We fear rejection, guilt, or confrontation. So we give in.

But at what cost?

- Your time gets stolen by other people's agendas
- Your focus is diluted
- Your values get compromised

- Your inner peace is disturbed

Saying "yes" out of fear is not kindness - it's self-abandonment.

## The Energy Equation

Your time, energy, and attention are **limited resources**. When you protect them, you grow. When you scatter them, you suffer.

Imagine you wake up each day with 100 energy points.

Every "yes" you say costs you points:

- 10 points for unnecessary meetings
- 15 points for social obligations you dread
- 20 points for helping someone who constantly drains you
- 25 points for tasks that aren't yours to carry

Suddenly, you're out of fuel - exhausted, unfocused, unhappy.

Saying "no" isn't rejection. It's redirection - of your energy, purpose, and peace.

## The Silent Power of Boundaries

Saying "no" is how you **build boundaries** - invisible fences that protect your time, heart, and mind.

Boundaries are not walls. They're doors you choose when to open.

They allow healthy people and experiences in - and keep the toxic or unnecessary out.

Examples of quiet, powerful boundaries:

- "I don't take calls after 9 p.m."
- "I'm not available on weekends."
- "I need to check my schedule and get back to you."
- "I'm focusing on something important right now."

Boundaries create space for joy, rest, and authenticity.

**Saying No Without Guilt**

Here's how to say no kindly but firmly:

1. **Be clear and direct.** "I won't be able to attend." "That's not something I can commit to right now."

2. **Don't over-explain.** You don't owe lengthy justifications. A simple reason (or none) is enough.

3. **Offer an alternative (if you want).**

    "I can't join, but I'd love to catch up next week."

    "I can't help with that, but I know someone who might."

4. **Stand your ground.** If someone pushes, stay calm and repeat: "I understand, but my answer is no."

Your peace is not up for negotiation.

**Where You Must Learn to Say No**

### ☑ To toxic people
You're not responsible for fixing, saving, or tolerating emotional vampires.

### ☑ To things that don't align with your values
Even if they look good or are expected of you - trust your gut.

### ☑ To your own impulses
Not every urge needs to be followed. Not every thought deserves action.

### ☑ To overcommitting
Saying yes to everything makes you mediocre at everything. Focus wins.

### ☑ To the pressure to be always available
Your time offline, in silence, or in solitude is sacred. Guard it.


**The Deeper Joy of Saying No**

When you say no to what doesn't serve you, you create space for what **does**:

- More time with people who uplift you
- More focus on your goals and growth
- More mental clarity and emotional stability
- More alignment between your values and actions

You stop living a life of reaction - and start living a life of **intention**.

Saying no is not a rejection of others. It's a declaration of *self-worth*.

## When You Say Yes, Make It a Sacred Yes

The goal isn't to become someone who always says no.

It's to become someone whose "yes" is **full**, **genuine**, and **joyful** - not forced, fearful, or fake.

When you say yes now:

- It's to things that nourish your soul
- It's to people who respect your boundaries
- It's to opportunities aligned with your purpose

That kind of yes brings happiness, not exhaustion.

---

## Final Thoughts

Self-control isn't just about resisting temptation - it's about **choosing wisely**. Sometimes the wisest choice is simply: **No.**

Every no that protects your peace is a yes to your happiness. And the more you practice it, the freer, lighter, and more authentic your life becomes.

In the next chapter, we'll explore how **mindfulness and self-control** work together - and how living fully in the present moment deepens joy and presence.

# Chapter 14

# Mindfulness & Self-Control – Living in the Moment

We live in a world full of distractions. Our minds jump between regrets of the past, worries about the future, and endless to-do lists.

It's easy to feel out of control - not just of our actions, but of our attention, our emotions, and our experience of life.

But what if the key to mastering self-control is not just more willpower... but more presence?

That's where mindfulness comes in.

Mindfulness is the art of paying attention - on purpose, in the present moment, without judgment.

And when paired with self-control, it becomes a superpower.

**The Connection Between Mindfulness & Self-Control**

At first glance, mindfulness and self-control seem like separate ideas. But in truth, they are deeply connected:

- Mindfulness helps you **notice your impulses**
- Self-control helps you **pause and choose your response**
- Together, they help you act with **intention**, not instinct

Imagine you feel the urge to scroll your phone, eat junk food, or react in anger.

A mindful person notices the urge without being consumed by it.

A self-controlled person *chooses* how to respond to it.

Mindfulness is the spotlight. Self-control is the steering wheel.

## Why We Lose Control: The Unconscious Mind

Most of our behaviors are automatic:

- We eat without tasting
- Speak without thinking
- React without understanding
- Live without noticing

This "autopilot mode" is the enemy of self-control.

Mindfulness turns off autopilot. It brings you back into the *driver's seat* of your life.

Every time you pause and become aware of what you're thinking, feeling, or doing, you **create a gap**. In that gap is the **power to choose**.

## Daily Mindfulness Practices to Strengthen Control

Here are simple ways to bring mindfulness into your daily life:

## 1. Mindful Breathing

Pause and take 3 deep breaths. Feel each inhale and exhale. Do this before eating, replying to messages, or entering a meeting.

This calms your nervous system and restores clarity.

## 2. Single-Tasking

Do one thing at a time - fully. Whether it's eating, walking, or talking - be there, 100%.

Multitasking divides your focus and drains your energy.

## 3. The STOP Technique

A quick tool for moments of stress:

- **S**: Stop what you're doing
- **T**: Take a deep breath
- **O**: Observe your thoughts, emotions, and sensations
- **P**: Proceed with awareness

This helps you respond wisely instead of reacting impulsively.

## 4. Mindful Moments

Choose one activity per day (like brushing your teeth or drinking tea) and do it *slowly, silently, fully present*.

Even 1 minute of mindfulness can rewire your brain over time.


## Living in the Present: The Gateway to Peace

So much suffering comes from **not being here**:

- Regret is about the past
- Anxiety is about the future
- But peace? It's only found *now*

When you're fully present:

- You eat with gratitude
- You listen with compassion
- You work with focus
- You rest with ease

Mindfulness allows you to experience life deeply, not just rush through it.

Presence turns the ordinary into sacred.

## Self-Control Is Easier When You're Present

When you're mindful:

- You *notice* the craving before it controls you
- You *feel* the anger rising, but don't let it explode
- You *catch* the negative thought before it spirals

Mindfulness helps you delay gratification, hold space for emotions, and align with your values.

Instead of being driven by desire or fear, you act from a place of centeredness.

## The Myth of Control vs. Flow

Ironically, true self-control isn't about tight control - it's about **inner alignment**.

You don't have to fight your emotions or suppress your desires. You just need to **witness them** with awareness.

Mindfulness doesn't judge your thoughts or feelings. It simply says, "I see you" and in that seeing, the intensity often fades.

This creates space for wiser action - not forced, but *flowing*.

## Mindfulness Is a Lifelong Practice

Like self-control, mindfulness isn't a one-time fix - it's a daily invitation.

There will be days when you forget to be present. You'll react, slip up, or feel overwhelmed.

That's okay.

Mindfulness says:

"Begin again. This moment is a fresh start."

No guilt. No drama. Just awareness and return.

Over time, this builds a **quiet inner strength** that anchors you in all situations.

**Final Thoughts**

Mindfulness isn't just meditation. It's a way of living - awake, aware, and alive. Combined with self-control, it helps you:

- Pause before reacting
- Choose peace over impulse
- Experience joy in the now

The present moment is the only place where change can happen. It's the only place where happiness is real.

So, breathe. Come back. This moment is waiting for you - and it's enough.


In the next and final chapter, we'll explore how to **redefine success and happiness** through the lens of self-mastery - and begin the lifelong journey of becoming the best version of yourself.

# Chapter 15

# Redefining Success – The Happiness of Self-Mastery

*"Success isn't something you chase-it's drawn to you through the qualities you develop within yourself."*

For years, society has taught us a formula:
**Success = Money + Status + Achievement**

We chase titles, trophies, and timelines. We measure ourselves against others. We hustle… and often feel hollow.

But what if this version of success is incomplete?

What if **true success** isn't about what you *get* - but about who you *become*?

Self-control leads to self-mastery and self-mastery is the foundation of lasting happiness and authentic success.

### The Traditional Model of Success: A Trap?

Our world rewards outward achievement:

- Degrees
- Promotions
- Accumulated wealth
- Social validation

And while none of these are bad, they come with a silent danger:

**You can win the world and still lose yourself.**

Many high achievers:

- Burn out
- Feel anxious or empty
- Constantly need more to feel "enough"

This is the **hedonic treadmill** - the more you get, the more you want.

Real success must be redefined - not as *external acquisition*, but *internal alignment*.


**What Is Self-Mastery?**

Self-mastery is the ability to:

- Understand yourself deeply
- Direct your thoughts and behaviors
- Align your life with your values
- Stay steady amid chaos
- Lead yourself before leading others

It doesn't mean perfection. It means progress with awareness.

You still feel temptation, anger, fear, doubt - but you're no longer ruled by them.

You become the captain of your inner world.

## Why Self-Control Is Central to Success

External success is built on inner discipline.

Think about it:

- You can't build wealth without resisting short-term pleasure
- You can't maintain health without saying no to unhealthy urges
- You can't nurture deep relationships without emotional regulation
- You can't pursue big goals without mental focus and consistency

In short:

**Self-control is the bridge between vision and reality.**

Without it, talent is wasted. Potential is lost. And joy is scattered.


## Redefining Success: A New Model

Let's build a new, more sustainable and fulfilling model of success - rooted in self-mastery.

### The Self-Mastery Success Formula:

- ☑ **Clarity** – Know what truly matters to you
- ☑ **Discipline** – Stay committed to those values
- ☑ **Presence** – Enjoy the journey, not just the outcome

- ☑ **Resilience** – Bounce back from setbacks
- ☑ **Contribution** – Use your gifts to uplift others

This path leads to not just success - but *significance*.

You become rich in:

- Purpose
- Peace
- Impact
- Integrity

**Signs You're Succeeding at Self-Mastery**

You'll know you're on the path when:

- You feel aligned between your thoughts, words, and actions
- You can pause before reacting
- You find joy in small things, not just big achievements
- You're able to say no without guilt
- You live by principles, not pressure
- Your inner peace isn't shaken by outside noise

This is quiet confidence. Deep contentment. Not flashy, but **powerful**.

## Letting Go of the Comparison Game

One of the fastest ways to lose happiness is to **compare your path to someone else's**.

Social media, society, and even family can trigger the belief that:

- You're not doing enough
- You're behind
- You should be more like them

But here's a gentle truth:

*You're not here to win anyone else's race. You're here to run your own - with grace.*

Self-mastery means:

- You define your own metrics for success
- You measure growth, not popularity
- You choose peace over pressure


## A Life of Purpose, Not Performance

When you live from self-mastery:

- You stop performing for approval
- You act from *purpose*, not people-pleasing
- You're driven by values, not vanity
- Your success feels *deep*, not just impressive

You realize:

The most successful life is one where your **soul feels safe inside your own skin.**

You no longer chase validation - because you've already found inner wholeness.

---

**Final Thoughts**

True success is *not* a destination - it's a byproduct of daily choices made with self-control, presence, and purpose.

It's waking up with:

- Peace in your heart
- Clarity in your mind
- Integrity in your actions

That's the happiness of self-mastery. And the beautiful thing is - it's available to everyone, right where they are.

You don't need to change the world to succeed. You just need to change your *inner world* - and the rest follows.


In the final chapter, we'll reflect on your journey and offer practical tools and inspiration for moving forward - toward a life of conscious growth and true fulfillment.

# Chapter 16

# Your Journey Forward – Becoming the Best Version of Yourself

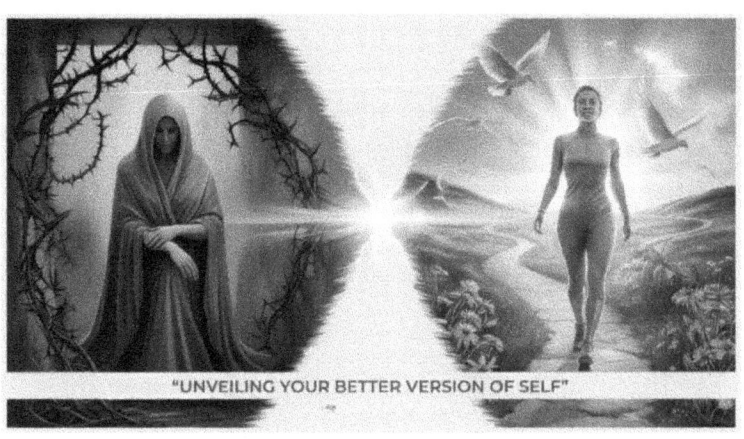

*"Each choice you make reflects the kind of person you're shaping yourself into."*

You've traveled far in these pages.

From understanding what self-control really means, to learning how it shapes your mind, emotions, habits, relationships, finances - and ultimately, your happiness.

Now the question becomes: Where do you go from here?

The path forward is not about achieving perfection. It's about becoming a little more intentional, a little more aligned, a little more awake - every single day.

This is your journey of self-mastery.
And it begins (again) now.

## The Ongoing Nature of Growth

Self-control is not a finish line. It's a **way of living**.

Some days you'll feel strong, focused, and clear. Other days you'll slip, stumble, or revert to old patterns.

That's okay.

Growth isn't linear - it spirals and every time you return to the path, you come back wiser, stronger, and more compassionate.

The key is to keep showing up. Keep choosing awareness over autopilot. Discipline over distraction. Peace over pressure.

That's where the transformation happens - in the small moments, repeated with care.

## Your Personal Compass: Values and Vision

To stay on course, you need a **compass** - something that guides your choices when temptations arise or motivation fades.

That compass is made of two things:

1. **Your Values** – What matters most to you
    - Integrity? Growth? Kindness? Freedom?

- Clarify your top 3–5 values and revisit them often

2. **Your Vision** – Who you want to become
    - Not just what you want to achieve, but who you want to *be*
    - Write it down. Speak it out loud. Live it through your choices.

When you align your actions with your values and vision, self-control becomes natural - because you're not forcing discipline... **you're living your truth.**


## Make It Practical: Daily Practices for the Journey

Here are simple, powerful tools to anchor your growth:

### 1. Daily Reflection (5 minutes at night)

Ask:

- Did I live with intention today?
- Where did I act out of impulse?
- What am I proud of? What can I improve?

This cultivates self-awareness - the foundation of self-control.

### 2. Morning Intention Setting (2 minutes)

Before starting your day, pause and ask:

- How do I want to show up today?
- What do I want to say *yes* to? What will I say *no* to?

Set one intention and carry it like a compass.

### 3. Habit Tracking

Choose 1–3 key habits that support your highest self. Track them daily - not for perfection, but for progress.

### 4. Mindfulness Check-ins

Set reminders to pause, breathe, and reconnect with the present. Just 1–2 minutes can shift your state.

### When You Fall Off Track (Because You Will)

You will mess up. You will lose focus. You will have lazy days or emotional slips.

That's part of the journey.

The important thing is how you **respond**:

- Don't shame yourself - learn from it
- Don't quit - recommit
- Don't wait for a perfect Monday - start now, in this moment

One conscious breath. One honest reflection. One mindful action.
That's all it takes to come home to yourself.

### Surround Yourself with Growth Energy

Your environment either supports or sabotages your self-control.

Curate your space, your inputs, and your relationships:

- Spend time with people who reflect the best in you
- Read and listen to things that uplift and challenge you
- Create physical spaces that inspire calm, not chaos
- Reduce exposure to temptations and noise

You don't have to do it alone. Growth is faster, deeper, and more joyful in *the community*.

## Celebrate Your Wins - Big and Small

Every time you:

- Pause instead of reacting
- Wake up and stick to your routine
- Say no to what drains you
- Stay present in the now
- Align with your values

Celebrate it. Smile. Journal. Acknowledge it.

These are not small things. They are *acts of self-respect*. They are proof that you are becoming the kind of person you admire.

## The Bigger Picture: Your Ripple Effect

As you grow in self-control and happiness, something beautiful happens:

You begin to inspire others - not by preaching, but simply by living.

- Your children, friends and coworkers observe your calm presence
- Your habits spark curiosity and admiration
- Your inner peace creates an outer impact

The best way to change the world is to first change yourself. And then - live, love, and lead from that place of clarity.

---

### Final Thoughts: The Adventure Continues

There is no final destination in self-mastery. Only deeper layers, brighter clarity and fuller joy.

You will evolve. You will face new tests and you will rise - because now, you know how.

You have the tools. You have the awareness. And most importantly - you have the **commitment to your own highest self**.

So, step forward.

Not as someone chasing happiness - but as someone who's learned to *create it*, *contain it*, and *live it*.

One choice at a time.

A Closing Reflection
You are not your impulses.
You are the space between
the impulse and the action.
You are not your past.
You are the author of every
new chapter you choose to write.
You are not broken.
You are becoming.
And your best - your calmest, clearest,
most powerful self - is not some
far-away dream.
It is already within you.

www.ingramcontent.com/pod-product-compliance
Lightning Source LLC
LaVergne TN
LVHW061554070526
838199LV00077B/7041